Paleo Bread

Delicious Healthy Muffins, Biscuits, and Gluten Free Bread Cookbook

Lucy Fast

Paleo Bread

Just to say Thank You for Purchasing this Book I want to give you a gift 100% absolutely FREE

A Copy of My Upcoming Special Report
"Paleo Pantry: The Beginner's Guide to What Should and Should NOT be in Your Paleo Kitchen"

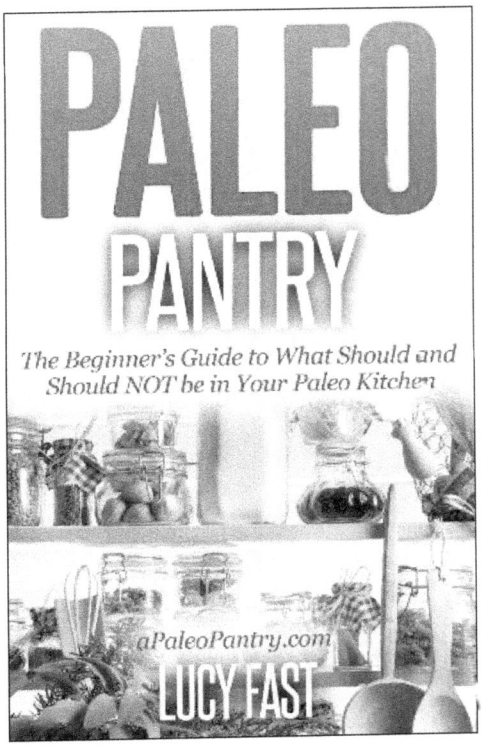

Go to www.aPaleoPantry.com to Reserve Your FREE Copy

Table of Contents

Introduction

I want to thank you and congratulate you for purchasing *"Paleo Bread: Delicious Healthy Muffins, Biscuits, and Gluten Free Bread Cookbook"*.

This book contains proven steps and strategies for how to welcome bread back into your life after the Paleo hiatus.
There is nothing better than bread in my opinion – not even chocolate! (OK maybe a Chocolate Croissant is best...)

But for me bread provides a complete well rounded sensory experience and there are few foods that can boast this. From getting elbow deep in sticky dough mixture, to kneading it into the perfect consistency, then watching a golden brown loaf rise in the oven, to the hearty, comforting aromas that fill the kitchen as it bakes. Then the piece de resistance – cutting open a piping hot loaf of homemade bread, slathering it in butter and honey and devouring a slice or 6! This for me is the ultimate decadent indulgence, because let's face it, who has time to bake bread from scratch when you can pop down to your local store and buy a perfectly sliced and pre-packaged loaf.

Well let me tell you, it's time to make time! You will thank me later.

One of the things that is most missed when people convert to the Paleo lifestyle is bread. Bread is convenient and tasty. We don't all have time at lunch to whip up a veggie stir fry or something else that's Paleo friendly AND tastes good. People end up having wistful fantasies about their favorite fillings lovingly encompassed between 2 slices of gluten-stuffed, clog your system, tummy bloating bread! And to be honest, there really could not be a worse Paleo cheat than succumbing to wheat based bread! The price you pay for days thereafter is just not worth it.

So I decided to don my super hero cape and swoop in to save you all from veering of the Paleo path (I'm kinda awesome like that!). I have put together an entire book on breads!!!

These recipes will fill that bread shaped hole in your life without all the ugly side effects. You can enjoy bread every day now, and all you have to do is dedicate just an hour every few days to get a fresh loaf baked – something I'm sure we all can manage if it means we can enjoy our sandwiches again!

For me, eating bread opens up a whole can of worms because I'm sort of an all or nothing kind of girl. So for those readers out there who are like me, I have not only catered to your every bread need – sweet, savory, every day and specialty – but I've also included some delicious biscuit and muffin recipes that will help keep your Paleo flag flying high! As an added bonus I have included a special chapter on international breads where you can learn how to make baguettes, croissants, pizza dough and the like, while still sticking to your Paleo principles 110%!

Remember, Paleo is not a life sentence to misery and deprivation, Paleo is an invitation to find alternatives that work for you! So without further ado, here are 38 fantastic, lip-smacking, hunger inducing bread, biscuit and muffin recipes to get you started! Have fun!

Thanks again for purchasing this book, I hope you enjoy it!

Lucy Fast

Sandwich Loafs, Buns and Wrappers

Sandwich Bread
Yields: **1 loaf**

<u>Ingredients</u>

¾ cup almond butter
½ cup apple cider vinegar
¼ cup coconut oil (melted)
¼ cup ground flax
¼ cup almond flour
¼ cup coconut flour
6 eggs
4 tablespoons honey
1 tsp baking soda
½ tsp sea salt

<u>Method</u>

1. Preheat the oven to 350°F and grease a loaf pan well with coconut oil then line the pan with parchment paper.
2. In a large bowl, whisk all the wet ingredients together.
3. In a separate bowl, mix the dry ingredients together.
4. Mix the dry ingredients into the wet ingredients and combine well.
5. Pour the batter into the greased pan and bake for 40 minutes or until a toothpick inserted into the center comes out clean.
6. Remove from the oven and allow the loaf to cool in the baking pan for about 10 min.
7. Remove the bread from the pan and leave to cool completely on a wire rack.
8. Store in an airtight container.

9. Slice and serve as desired with your favorite sandwich fillings.

Paleo Bread

Best Basic Breakfast Bread
Yields: **1 loaf**

Ingredients

½ cup almond butter
4 tablespoons honey
2 tablespoons cinnamon
2 eggs
1 teaspoon finely grated orange zest
1 teaspoon vanilla extract
½ teaspoon nutmeg
¼ teaspoon baking soda

Method

1. Preheat oven to 325°F.
2. Beat the almond butter until it is creamy, then whisk in eggs, honey and vanilla extract.
3. Now add nutmeg, baking soda, orange zest and cinnamon and mix together well
4. Pour the mixture into a well-greased loaf pan
5. Place in the oven and bake for 15 minutes or until a toothpick inserted in the center comes out clean.
6. Remove from the oven and allow to cool down, then slice and serve.
7. Store any left overs in an airtight container.

Easy Everyday Bread
Yields: **1 loaf**

<u>Ingredients</u>

5 eggs
2 cups almond flour
¼ cup ground sunflower seeds
2 tablespoons flax seeds - ground
2 tablespoons raw honey
1 tablespoon apple cider vinegar
1 tablespoon olive oil
½ tsp baking soda

<u>Method</u>

1. Preheat the oven at 350°F and grease a loaf pan well with a little olive oil.
2. Mix the dry ingredients together in a bowl.
3. Whisk the wet ingredients together in a separate bowl.
4. Pour the wet bowl into the dry one and stir well to combine.
5. Pour the batter into well-greased loaf pan.
6. Place into the oven and bake for 30 min or until a toothpick inserted in the center comes out clean.
7. Allow to cool for about 2 hours, then store in an airtight container until needed.
8. To serve, spread with a little Paleo mayonnaise or almond butter and your choice of delicious fillings.

Sourdough Bread
Yields: **1 loaf**

Ingredients

2 cups cashews – chopped into pieces
½ cup + 1 tablespoon water
2 large eggs, separated
1 egg yolk + 1 tablespoon water for the egg wash
½ tsp baking soda
¼ tsp sea salt
Olive oil
Probiotic capsules (enough to equal 30 billion probiotic strains)
*Note – probiotic capsules are available at most health food stores. They come in different strains per capsule

Method

1. Place the cashew nuts into the food processor and pulse until they are ground into a fine powder.
2. Add the water and probiotic powder and pulse until the mixture is thick. This might take some time depending on your blender, so you need to be patient.
3. Transfer the mixture to an airtight container and leave it overnight for the probiotic strains to culture.
4. Next day - Preheat the oven to 300°F and grease a loaf pan well with olive oil and line it with some parchment paper.
5. Transfer the cashew mixture into a large bowl. Add the 2 egg yolks and a tablespoon of water and beat with a hand held beater till very smooth, then add baking soda and salt to the mixture and stir well.
6. Rinse the beaters completely and dry them off.
7. Wash the egg beaters thoroughly and dry them off.
8. Now beat the egg whites until they are soft and fluffy.

9. Gently fold in the egg whites into the cashew mixture. Keep mixing gently until egg whites are no longer visible.
10. Place the batter into the prepared pan.
11. Prepare an egg wash by mixing an egg yolk with water and then gently brush the egg wash on the top of the batter. This will make a nice crunchy crust on top.
12. Bake for 40 min or until a toothpick inserted in the center comes out clean.
13. After 40 min increase the oven to 375°F and bake for an additional 5 – 10 min, or until the top is golden brown and crispy.
14. Remove from oven and allow to cool before slicing.
15. Store the left overs in an airtight container and serve as desired.

Dinner Rolls

Yields: **10 rolls** (depending on how big you want them)

<u>Ingredients</u>

1 cup arrowroot flour
½ cup almond flour
¼ cup coconut flour
½ cup of warm water
½ cup olive oil
1 egg – beaten
1 teaspoon salt

<u>Method</u>

1. Preheat oven to 350°F and line a baking tray with parchment paper.
2. Mix arrowroot flour, salt and ¼ cup almond flour in a bowl
3. Pour in the olive oil and warm water. Stir well.
4. Add the beaten egg and continue mixing well, then add the rest of the flours.
5. If the mixture is too runny add one or two more tablespoons of coconut flour and if it is too stiff add a little more water. (Dough must be soft but not sticky.)
6. Use a large spoon to place 2 scoops of the mixture onto a lightly floured surface. Roll the mixture into a ball. You should end up with about 10 balls.
7. Place each roll onto the baking tray.
8. Place the tray into the oven and bake for about 35 minutes until golden brown.
9. Serve nice and warm

Garlic Knots
Yields: **6 garlic knots**

<u>Ingredients</u>

½ cup of water
½ cup olive oil
¾ cup tapioca flour
¼ cup almond flour
1 egg
1 teaspoon salt
1 teaspoon crushed garlic
½ teaspoon Italian herbs

<u>Method</u>

1. Place the olive oil, water and sea salt into a pan and bring to the boil.
2. Remove from the heat and add the garlic and tapioca flour.
3. Mix thoroughly and let the mixture set for 5 minutes.
4. Add the Italian herbs and egg and mix well.
5. Now stir in the almond flour.
6. Place dough onto a lightly floured surface and knead for a few minutes.
7. Divide the dough into 12 equal balls, then roll each one into a long rope.
8. Take two ropes of dough and knot them together, then place them onto a well-greased baking tray. Repeat till all the dough is finished.
9. Bake them in a 350° F oven for 40 minutes or until nicely golden.
10. Take them out and let cool.
11. These are amazing - enjoy!

Cauliflower Breadsticks

<u>Ingredients</u>

1 head of cauliflower
1 tablespoon garlic powder
1 tablespoon paprika
½ teaspoon red pepper flakes
2 eggs
Salt and pepper to taste

<u>Method</u>

1. Boil the whole cauliflower until it is soft.
2. Place it into a blender, pulse it until it is smooth and then leave it to cool down.
3. Once cooled add the garlic powder, paprika, red pepper flakes and eggs, then season with salt and pepper.
4. Grease a baking tray with a little olive oil.
5. Place the mixture into the tray and pat it down in an even layer until it is ¼ - ½ inch thick.
6. Place the baking tray into a 350° F oven for 20 minutes or until the cauliflower turns golden brown and the edges begin to crisp.
7. To make the sticks even crispier cut it into thin slices and flip them and place them back into the oven just to brown the other side.
8. Allow to cool and enjoy.
9. These are totally addictive – expect to eat the whole batch in one sitting.

Herb Focaccia Bread
Yields: **6-8 slices**

<u>Ingredients</u>

4 eggs
¼ cup almond flour
¼ cup coconut cream
1 tablespoon crushed garlic
1 teaspoon parsley
1 teaspoon thyme
1 teaspoon basil
1 teaspoon oregano
½ teaspoon baking soda
Olive oil for drizzling
Course sea salt (for topping)

<u>Method</u>

1. Preheat the oven to 375°F
2. Beat eggs and coconut cream until smooth.
3. In a bowl, mix almond flour, herbs and baking soda together.
4. Add the egg mixture to the dry ingredients and mix well.
5. Grease a pie pan well and spread the batter into the pan.
6. Drizzle olive oil over the batter, then scatter the crushed garlic and finish off with a sprinkling of course sea salt. Using your fingers press the salt and garlic lightly into the batter.
7. Place in oven for 20 minutes or until the top is golden brown.
8. Remove from the oven and cool on a wire rack before serving.
9. Finger licking good!

Tasty Tortillas
Yields: **8 tortillas**

<u>Ingredients</u>

1 cup tapioca flour
½ cup water
½ cup flax meal
3 eggs
4 egg whites
2 tablespoons baking powder
1 tablespoon olive oil
½ teaspoon coarse sea salt
Olive oil for frying

<u>Method</u>

1. Whisk eggs, egg whites and water into a bowl.
2. Drizzle 1 tablespoon of olive oil in while whisking.
3. In a separate bowl mix all the dry ingredients together well.
4. Combine the dry ingredients with the wet ingredients and mix well. The batter will be thin and runny like a pancake batter. If it doesn't run easily, add a little more water.
5. Heat a little olive oil in a non-stick pan over a medium-high heat and pour 1/3 cup of batter into the hot pan.
6. Coat the bottom of the pan with batter and cook for about 2 minutes on each side.
7. Allow to cool, then stuff them full of your favorite fillings.
8. Enjoy!

Hamburger Buns
Yields: **8 buns**

<u>Ingredients</u>

8 tablespoons almond flour
4 eggs
4 tablespoons melted coconut oil
1 teaspoon baking powder
½ tsp sea salt
Sesame seeds/poppy seeds for topping

<u>Method</u>

1. Preheat the oven to 350°F
2. Using a fork mix the almond flour, baking powder and sea salt in a large bowl.
3. In a separate bowl, beat eggs until the eggs are fluffy and add the coconut oil. Mix well.
4. Pour egg-oil mixture into the flour mixture and stir them together well.
5. Line your baking pan with parchment paper and grease the paper with a little coconut oil.
6. Divide the dough into 8 equal sized portions and place on the baking tray.
7. Sprinkle sesame seeds and/or poppy seeds on top and bake for 15 minutes.
8. Allow to cool before serving.
9. Top with delicious Paleo hamburger patties and your choice of condiments and garnish.
10. Superb!

Paleo Bread

Quick and Easy Individual Wrap
Yields: **1 - 2 wraps** (depending on size)

<u>Ingredients</u>

2 eggs
3 tablespoons olive oil
2 tablespoons almond flour
Pinch of salt

<u>Method</u>

1. Beat the eggs well with a beater.
2. Add flour, olive oil and salt together and mix well. The mixture must be quite runny like a pancake mixture.
3. Heat a little bit of olive oil in a pan and pour enough batter in to cover the bottom of the pan.
4. Cook on a medium- high heat for a few minutes then flip and cook the other side.
5. Serve immediately with your choice of fillings

Note – this is a basic recipe. Jazz it up to your personal taste by adding herbs and seasonings. Great options to add are garlic powder, paprika, onion powder, red pepper flakes, cumin, Italian herbs and even curry powder for something unusual.

Caveman Crepes

Yields: **6 crepes**

Ingredients

2 tablespoons olive oil
1 tablespoon arrowroot powder
4 teaspoons coconut milk
4 large eggs

Method

1. Place all the ingredients together in a bowl and blend well.
2. Heat up a non-stick pan over a medium- high heat. (Use a crepe pan if you have)
3. Grease your pan lightly with olive oil before making each crepe.
4. Pour about 3 table spoons of batter in to the frying pan and gently coat the bottom of the pan with batter (the batter must be quite thin)
5. Once the sides of the crepe start to lift softly release the rest using a spatula.
6. Once the crepe has lifted gently flip it over and brown the other side.
7. Now it is ready to be eaten or filled.
8. Choose from a variety of sweet and savory fillings to make uniquely scrumptious crepes every time!

Paleo Sweet Breads

Cinnamon Rolls
Yield: **9 rolls**

<u>Ingredients for the Rolls</u>
2 cups almond flour
¼ cup coconut oil – softened but not melted
½ cup water
4 tablespoons honey
1 tablespoon vanilla extract
2 eggs
½ teaspoon salt

<u>Ingredients for the Filling</u>
½ cup raisins
¼ cup maple syrup
2 tablespoons coconut oil
2 tablespoons cinnamon

<u>Ingredients for the Topping</u>
½ cup nuts of your choice - chopped
¼ cup maple syrup
¼ cup coconut oil – softened but not melted
1 tablespoon vanilla extract

<u>Method</u>

1. Place all the ingredients for the rolls into a bowl and knead until the mixture forms a smooth dough.
2. Place the dough into the fridge for 15 minutes.
3. Meanwhile, make the filling – mix the softened coconut oil and maple syrup together and set aside.
4. Remove the dough from the fridge and roll it out into a large rectangle shape of about ½ an inch thickness.

5. Spread the coconut oil and maple syrup over the dough, then sprinkle on the cinnamon and raisins.
6. Roll the rectangle up so it forms a log and then keep rolling it gently to smooth it out on all sides.
7. Cut the log into 2 inch thick sections and lay them flat onto a parchment lined baking tray.
8. Bake in a 350° F oven for 20 minutes.
9. Remove from the oven and allow to cool for 10 minutes.
10. While the rolls are cooling, mix all the topping ingredients except the nuts together in a bowl and drizzle the mixture over the cinnamon rolls, then sprinkle the chopped nuts on top.
11. Left overs – I think not!

Banana Bread
Yields: **1 loaf**

<u>Ingredients</u>

1 cup almond flour
¼ cup raw honey
3 eggs
3 bananas – the riper the better (brown is OK too)
2 teaspoons olive oil
1 teaspoon baking soda
1 teaspoon baking powder
1 teaspoon vanilla extract
1 teaspoon cinnamon
½ tsp salt
¼ teaspoon nutmeg

<u>Method</u>

1. Preheat oven to 350°F
2. Prepare a loaf pan by greasing it well with olive oil.
3. In a bowl whisk baking soda, baking powder, salt, cinnamon, nutmeg and flour.
4. In a separate bowl mix all the wet ingredients.
5. Gently add wet ingredients to the dry ingredients and stir. Be careful you do not over mix
6. Pour the batter into the loaf pan and bake it for 50 minutes or until the middle of the cake has set. You can check the center of the loaf by inserting a tooth pick into the loaf and if it comes out clean and dry the loaf is done.
7. Allow the loaf to cool for about 15 minutes inside the pan, then tip out the loaf onto a wire rack and allow to cool completely.
8. Serve and enjoy

Note – you can jazz up this recipe with some chopped nuts, raisins and/or chocolate chips or you could even bake it with some banana slices drizzled with maple syrup on top – the end result is a deliciously caramelized topping! YUM!

Easy Pumpkin Loaf
Yields: **1 loaf**

Ingredients

1 ½ cups almond flour
½ cup olive oil
½ cup pumpkin puree
¼ cup pumpkin seeds
4 large eggs
2 tablespoons honey
3 teaspoons pumpkin pie spice
½ teaspoon salt
½ teaspoon baking powder
½ teaspoon cinnamon

Method

1. Preheat the oven to 350°F and grease a loaf pan well with some olive oil.
2. Mix all dry ingredients together.
3. In another bowl mix the eggs and olive oil together.
4. Add pumpkin puree and honey and mix again.
5. Slowly add the dry ingredients into the wet ingredients and mix well until well combined.
6. Pour the batter into the pan and place into the oven
7. Bake for 40 minutes.
8. Allow to cool on a wire rack, then slice and serve.
9. This is amazing!

Chocolate Zucchini Bread

Yields: **1 loaf**

<u>Ingredients</u>

1 ½ cups almond flour
1 ½ cups cocoa powder
1 cup zucchini – finely grated
½ cup walnuts – chopped
½ cup chocolate chips
¼ cup sweet potato puree
¼ cup olive oil
1 egg
4 tablespoons raw honey
1 tablespoon apple cider vinegar
1 teaspoon vanilla extract
1 teaspoon baking soda
1 teaspoon ground cinnamon

<u>Method</u>

1. Preheat oven to 350°F and grease a loaf pan well with olive oil.
2. Mix almond flour with baking soda, cocoa powder and cinnamon.
3. In a separate bowl, beat the egg then add sweet potato, olive oil, vanilla, raw honey and apple cider vinegar. Mix well.
4. Stir in grated zucchini, chopped walnuts and chocolate chips
5. Pour the batter into the loaf pan
6. Bake for 40 minutes.
7. Take out the pan and allow to cool before cutting and serving.
8. This is a totally decadent treat!

Savory Biscuits

Sweet Potato, Bacon and Chive Biscuits
Yields: **8 biscuits**

<u>Ingredients</u>

1 large sweet potato
3 eggs - beaten
8 strips of bacon - diced
4 tablespoons chives – chopped
3 tablespoons almond flour
1 teaspoon baking powder
Salt and pepper to taste

<u>Method</u>

1. Preheat oven to 415°F
2. Poke holes into sweet potato with a fork and place it onto a baking tray.
3. Put the potato into the oven for 40 minutes or until the potato is soft, then set it aside to cool.
4. Cook the bacon in a non-stick pan until it is brown and crispy. Drain fat off and set aside for later and place the bacon on a paper towel lined plate.
5. Once the sweet potato is cooled, scoop out the flesh and mash it well.
6. Add the egg to the mash potato and mix well.
7. Now add the bacon fat and mix well again.
8. Add all dry ingredients to the sweet potato and mix.
9. Finally add the cooked diced bacon and chives. Make sure all the ingredients are thoroughly combined.
10. Line a baking tray with parchment paper.
11. Using a large spoon place blobs of the mixture on to the tray.

12. Place into oven and bake for 25 minutes or until they are golden brown and crispy.
13. Once cooked take them out of the oven and allow to cool.
14. Now enjoy!
15. Highly addictive – you have been warned!

Herb and Onion Biscuits
Yields: **8 biscuits**

<u>Ingredients</u>

¼ cup onion flakes
6 tablespoons almond flour
6 tablespoons olive oil
6 tablespoons almond milk
2 eggs
2 garlic cloves, finely chopped
1 teaspoon dried mixed herbs
½ teaspoon apple cider vinegar
¼ teaspoon baking soda

<u>Method</u>

1. Preheat oven to 350°F and line a large baking tray with parchment paper.
2. Mix the almond flour, olive oil, onion, garlic, eggs, herbs and almond milk together well
3. Allow the mixture to sit for 5 min or so. This allows the batter to rise a bit.
4. Now mix in baking soda and vinegar.
5. Using a tablespoon, drop scoops of batter onto the baking tray.
6. Bake for 15 minutes. The biscuits should be soft but make sure that they are cooked through.
7. Allow to cool completely before serving and handle them gently because they are very crumbly when they are taken out of the oven. Allowing them to cool will give the biscuits the opportunity to harden.
8. Gobble up these delicious savory biscuits.

Pumpkin and Flax Biscuits
Yields: **12 biscuits**

Ingredients

1 cup coconut flour
½ cup ghee - melted
½ cup pumpkin seeds - chopped
¼ cup flax seeds
1 tablespoon apple cider vinegar
1 teaspoon baking soda
½ teaspoon sea salt
5 large eggs

Method

1. Preheat the oven to 350°F
2. Mix the coconut flour, baking soda and salt together well.
3. In a different bowl whisk the eggs together with the apple cider vinegar.
4. Add the flour mixture and beat well with hand held beater. The mixture will become thick.
5. Add the ghee and mix well.
6. Fold in the pumpkin seeds and the flax seeds.
7. Spoon the mixture onto a well-greased baking tray. You should be able to make 12 biscuits balls.
8. Place in oven for 15 minutes or until the tops are slightly browned
9. Take out oven and allow to cool.
10. Eat and Enjoy!

Garlic and Parsley Biscuits
Yields: 8 biscuits

<u>Ingredients</u>

¼ cup almond flour
¼ cup coconut cream
2 tablespoons coconut flour
2 tablespoons coconut oil
1 tablespoon crushed garlic
1 teaspoon baking soda
¼ teaspoon sea salt
1 egg
Olive oil and freshly chopped parsley for topping

<u>Method</u>

1. Preheat oven to 350°F and grease a baking tray well with olive oil.
2. Mix all the dry ingredients together.
3. Add the rest of the ingredients and mix well with a wooden spoon.
4. Using a large spoon scoop out the dough onto the greased baking tray making 8 even sized blobs. Leave 2 inches between biscuits.
5. Place in the oven and bake for 15 minutes.
6. Take out the oven and brush a bit of olive oil over the tops of the biscuits and then sprinkle a little parsley over them.
7. Serve warm and enjoy. YUM

Note – you can substitute any herbs to sprinkle on top for variation.

Cookies and Bars (or Sweet Biscuits)

"Jam" Thumbprint Biscuits
Yields: **12 biscuits**

<u>Ingredients</u>

3 cups almond flour
½ cup + 4 tablespoons honey
½ cup coconut oil, melted
1 tablespoon vanilla extract
½ tsp baking soda
¼ tsp salt
6 strawberries - chopped

<u>Method</u>

1. Pre heat oven to 350°F and line a baking tray with parchment paper.
2. Place the strawberries and 4 tablespoons of honey together in a bowl and then microwave on high for 3 minutes.
3. Remove the mixture from the microwave and mash with a fork. This will be your "jam".
4. Mix all dry ingredients together.
5. Mix all wet ingredients together.
6. Now add the wet ingredients to the dry and mix together.
7. Form into ½ inch size balls and flatten lightly with the back of a spoon.
8. Bake for 8 minutes.
9. Remove from the oven and indent the dough with your thumb. Take care not to burn!
10. Fill the hole with strawberry jam.

11. Place back into the oven for 5 minutes or until the biscuits are golden brown.
12. Allow to cool on a wire rack.
13. Once cooled eat and enjoy!

Amazing Chocolate Biscuits
Yields: **9 biscuits**

<u>Ingredients</u>

1 cup almond flour
1 tablespoons cocoa powder
4 teaspoons grated dark chocolate
3 teaspoons coconut oil – melted
2 teaspoons vanilla extract
2 teaspoons honey
¼ teaspoon baking soda
¼ teaspoon salt

<u>Method</u>

1. Preheat oven to 350°F and grease a baking pan well with olive oil.
2. Mix almond flour, baking soda, cocoa powder and salt.
3. Mix in coconut oil, vanilla and honey.
4. Add water 1 teaspoon at a time to bring the mixture together.
5. Slowly stir in the chocolate chips into the batter.
6. Pour the batter in the baking pan and place into the oven.
7. Bake for 15 minutes or until the biscuit is golden brown.
8. Cut the biscuit into squares and allow to cool in the pan for 10 minutes.
9. Eat and enjoy!

Thin Mints
Yields: **20 thins**

<u>Ingredients</u>

1 ½ cup almond flour
1 ½ cups dark chocolate chunks
¼ cup honey
2 tablespoons cocoa powder
2 teaspoons peppermint extract
2 teaspoons vegan shortening
1 teaspoon coconut flour
¼ teaspoon baking soda

<u>Method</u>

1. Mix almond flour, cocoa powder, coconut flour and baking soda together.
2. Add shortening, 1 tsp peppermint extract and honey and mix very well until it forms a dough.
3. Place the dough in between two pieces of parchment paper and roll out dough until 1/8 inch thick.
4. Place in the freezer for 15 minutes.
5. Preheat the oven to 350°F
6. Using a round cookie cutter cut out the dough till there is no dough left
7. Place cut out biscuits on a parchment lined baking tray.
8. Place the tray into the oven and bake for 5 minutes.
9. Melt the chocolate and peppermint extract in a pot over a medium- high heat.
10. Dip each biscuit into the chocolate and place on a plate.
11.

12. Freeze the biscuits for 1 hour.
13. Eat and enjoy.

Chocolate and Cranberry Biscotti
Yields: **24 biscotti**

<u>Ingredients</u>

½ cup pecan nuts – roughly chopped
½ cups honey
½ cup dried cranberries
½ cup dark chocolate chips
2 eggs
1 tablespoon vanilla extract
¼ teaspoon sea salt
½ teaspoon baking soda

<u>Method</u>

1. Preheat oven to 325°F
2. In a big bowl mix honey, eggs and vanilla extract and mix well with a hand blender till the mixture is fluffy.
3. In a different bowl, mix almond flour, baking soda and salt together then add to the first bowl and mix until a dough forms.
4. Gently fold the pecan nuts, cranberries and chocolate pieces into the mixture.
5. Place the dough onto a lightly floured surface. Roll the dough into a log shape about 12 inch long and 3 inch thick.
6. Place the dough log onto a parchment lined baking tray and bake in the oven for 30 minutes.
7. Remove from the oven and allow to cool for 20 minutes.
8. Place the biscuit log on to a chopping board and cut ½ inch slices and place them back onto the baking tray with the parchment paper.
9. Bake for a further 15 minutes or until golden brown.

10. Take out of oven and allow to cool for 2C min so that the biscotti get nice and crunchy.

Savory Muffins

Spicy Egg Muffins
Yields: **12 muffins**

<u>Ingredients</u>

12 eggs
½ cup roasted green chilies - diced
4 spring onions - finely chopped
2 teaspoons cilantro - finely chopped
½ teaspoon sea salt
¼ tablespoon black pepper

<u>Method</u>

1. Pre heat oven to 350°F and lightly grease your muffin tray with olive oil.
2. In a medium bowl mix roasted green chilies, cilantro, spring onions, salt and pepper together.
3. Place the mixture into the muffin cups evenly, and leave to one side.
4. In a large bowl lightly beat your eggs. Pour the eggs over the top of the chili mixture in the muffin cups. Pour until the cups are ¾ full.
5. Place the baking tray into the oven and bake for 25 minutes or until the eggs are cooked.
6. Serve warm. YUMMY!

Italian Pizza Muffins

Yields: **12 muffins**

<u>Ingredients</u>

4 ½ cups almond flour
½ cup coconut oil – melted
½ cup baby spinach leaves - chopped
12 tablespoons water
4 tablespoons ground flax seed
1 tablespoon parsley – finely chopped
1 tablespoon garlic powder
8 slices bacon - cooked and finely chopped
8 thin slices of salami - diced

<u>Method</u>

1. Preheat oven to 375°F and place paper cup holders into your muffin tray.
2. Mix flax seed and water together and allow to stand for a minute or so.
3. Mix the rest of the ingredients together.
4. Scoop the batter evenly into each cupcake holder.
5. Bake for 45 minutes or until a toothpick inserted into the center comes out clean.
6. Serve warm and enjoy!

Garlic and Herb Muffins
Yields: **12 muffins**

<u>Ingredients</u>

2 ½ cups almond flour
1 ½ cups mixed herbs – finely chopped
4 large eggs
2 egg whites
6 tablespoons garlic infused olive oil
¾ teaspoon baking soda
Salt and pepper to taste

<u>Method</u>

1. Preheat oven 350°F and line the muffin baking tray with paper cup holders.
2. Mix almond flour and baking soda in a large mixing bowl and season with salt and pepper.
3. In a different bowl, mix olive oil, eggs and egg whites until they go frothy.
4. Pour the egg mixture into the bowl with the dry ingredients and mix well using a hand held beater.
5. Whilst mixing slowly add the mixed herbs.
6. Now evenly divide the batter into the paper cup holders and place the tray into the oven.
7. Bake for 30 minutes or until a toothpick inserted into the center comes out clean.
8. Remove from baking tray and allow to cool on wire rack for 20 min.
9. Devour!

Mini Olive and Rosemary Muffins
Yields: **12 -16 mini muffins or 6 large muffins**

Ingredients

16 pitted black olives
1 small garlic clove - finely chopped
6 sprigs rosemary
4 large eggs
4 tablespoons olive oil
¼ cup arrowroot powder
¼ cup almond flour
¼ teaspoon baking powder

Method

1. Preheat the oven to 375°F and place mini cupcake holders into a mini muffin tray. If you don't have a mini muffin tray just place 6 cupcake holders into a big muffin tray.
2. In a bowl mix arrowroot, almond flour, and baking powder together.
3. Finely chop olives, garlic and rosemary with a knife.
4. In a separate bowl whisk together olive oil and eggs and mix well.
5. Add the olive oil and egg mixture to the dry ingredients and mix very well.
6. Add the chopped garlic mix and combine well.
7. Pour the batter evenly into the cupcake holders and place tray into the oven.
8. Bake for 15 minutes or until the tops are slightly golden.
9. Remove from oven and place the muffins on to a wire rack to cool.
10. Dive in and enjoy!

Sweet Muffins

"White Chocolate" and Strawberry Muffins
Yields: **10 muffins**

<u>Ingredients</u>

1 banana
1 ½ cups almond flour
1 cup strawberries - chopped
½ cup honey
¼ cup coconut oil – melted
¼ cup cocoa butter - melted
2 eggs
1 teaspoon baking soda
½ teaspoon vanilla essence

<u>Method</u>

1. Preheat oven to 320°F and grease a muffin tray well with olive oil.
2. Beat coconut oil, banana, honey, egg, vanilla and cocoa butter together well.
3. In another bowl mix almond flour and baking soda together. Make sure that there are no lumps.
4. Now add wet and the dry ingredients together and mix.
5. Slowly fold the strawberries into the batter.
6. Evenly divide the batter into the muffin baking tray.
7. Place the baking tray into oven and bake for 25 minutes.
8. Allow to cool on a wire rack and then tuck in.

Amaretto Muffins
Yields: **10 muffins**

<u>Ingredients</u>

1 cup coconut milk
1 cup coconut flour
1 cup frozen raspberries
½ cup granulated stevia
2 teaspoons baking powder
1 teaspoon almond essence
3 eggs

<u>Method</u>

1. Preheat oven to 350°F and place paper cup holders into a muffin tray.
2. Mix all the ingredients excluding the raspberries together until you get a smooth batter.
3. Fold in the raspberries
4. Pour the batter evenly into the muffin cups and place into the oven.
5. Bake for 30 min or until the tops are golden in color.
6. They are delicious when hot.
7. Easy as pie!

Maple Nut Crunch Muffins
Yields: **12 muffins**

<u>Ingredients for the Muffins</u>
1 banana
6 pitted dates
4 eggs
4 tablespoons maple syrup
¼ cup coconut oil - melted
3 tablespoons almond flour
1 teaspoon baking powder
1 teaspoon baking soda
2 tablespoons cocoa powder
1 teaspoon cinnamon

<u>Ingredients for the Topping</u>
1 cup mixed nuts - chopped
2 ½ tablespoons almond flour
A sprinkle of cinnamon
2 tablespoons maple syrup

<u>Method</u>

1. Preheat the oven to 350°F and grease the muffin tray well.
2. Put banana and dates into a blender and make a puree. Ensure that the dates are fully chopped up.
3. Add eggs, maple syrup and coconut oil and blend.
4. Now add the almond flour and cocoa powder and mix well
5. Add baking soda, baking powder and cinnamon and blend.
6. In a bowl add all the topping ingredients and mix well until all nuts are well coated
7. Using a large spoon, spoon the batter into the muffin tray evenly.
8. Place a heaped tablespoon of topping on each muffin. Ensure that the whole top of the muffin is covered.

9. Put muffin tray into the oven and bake for 40 minutes or until a toothpick inserted in the center comes out clean.
10. Let cool for 20 min. serve warm and enjoy.
11. These are scrumptious!

Tea Cakes
Yields: **12 muffins**

<u>Ingredients</u>

¼ cup coconut oil - melted
¼ cup honey
½ cup almond milk
4 eggs
1 ½ cups almond flour
2 teaspoons baking powder
½ teaspoon salt

<u>Method</u>

1. Preheat oven to 350°F and grease a muffin tray well with olive oil.
2. Mix the wet ingredients together in a bowl.
3. Mix the dry ingredients together in a bowl.
4. Pour the wet ingredients into the dry ones and stir well to combine.
5. Evenly divide the batter into the muffin tray and bake for 30 minutes. To test if the muffins are ready, insert a toothpick into the muffin and pull it out. If the toothpick is clean the muffins are ready.
6. Take out of the oven and allow to cool on a wire rack.
7. Eat and enjoy!

International Breads

Baguettes
Yields: **1 baguette**

Ingredients

1 ¾ cups almond flour
½ cup boiling water
2 eggs
4 tablespoons finely ground flax seeds
4 tablespoons raw honey
2 tablespoons apple cider vinegar
1 tablespoon rosemary
3 teaspoons baking powder
1 teaspoon salt

Method

1. Mix all the ingredients together in a large bowl until a dough forms. The dough will be a bit sticky, but it is manageable.
2. Line your French bread pan with some parchment paper and place the dough into it.
3. Grease your hands with some olive oil and smooth the top of the dough in the pan. This also helps the bread to bake nice and golden.
4. Bake in a 350° F oven for 1 hour, then remove from the oven and allow to cool on a wire rack before slicing.
5. This is the perfect accompaniment to a delicious Paleo soup.
6. Enjoy!

Soft Pretzels
Yields: **10 pretzels**

<u>Ingredients</u>

1 cup almond flour`.
½ cup tapioca flour
½ cup water
½ cup olive oil
1 egg
2 tablespoons ghee - melted
2 tablespoons apple cider vinegar
1 tablespoon coarse salt – or more to taste
1 teaspoon salt
½ teaspoon baking powder
½ teaspoon baking soda

<u>Method</u>

1. Place the water, olive oil, apple cider vinegar and ½ teaspoon salt into a saucepan and bring it to the boil.
2. Remove the pan from the heat and stir in the tapioca flour until you get a paste.
3. Add the baking soda and baking powder and keep stirring while the mixture froths.
4. Add in the almond flour and egg and keep mixing until a dough begins to form.
5. Knead the dough on a lightly floured surface until it is smooth.
6. Divide the dough into 10 equal portions and then roll each one out into a log shape.
7. Form the log into a pretzel shape and place on a parchment lined baking tray.
8. Brush the tops of the pretzels with melted ghee and sprinkle over the coarse salt.

9. Bake at 350° F for 30 minutes or until the pretzels are golden brown.
10. Allow to cool before getting stuck in (hard I know!)

Irish Soda Bread
Yield: **1 loaf**

<u>Ingredients</u>

4 cups almond flour
3 cups almond milk
½ cup raisins
1 egg – beaten
3 tablespoons apple cider vinegar
1 teaspoon dill seeds
1 teaspoon anise seeds
1 teaspoon baking powder
1 teaspoon baking soda
1 teaspoon sea salt

<u>Method</u>

1. Preheat oven to 375°F and grease a loaf pan well with olive oil.
2. Plump up raisins by pouring boiling water over them and leaving them for about 10 min.
3. Mix flour, salt, dill seeds, anise seeds, baking soda and baking powder in a large bowl.
4. Add the egg, almond milk and apple cider vinegar and mix well.
5. Take the raisins out of water, chop them finely and add them to the dough. Ensure the dough is firm enough to hold shape, if not add more flour.
6. Knead the dough on a lightly floured surface for about 5 minutes, then place it into the prepared pan.
7. Use a knife to cut a cross on the top of the dough.
8. Place in the oven and bake for about 1 hour.
9. Once cooked, place it on to a wire rake to cool. You will know it is cooked when you tap the surface and the bread makes a hollow sound.

Croissants
Yields: **18 croissants**

<u>Ingredients</u>

1 egg white (for brushing)
2 eggs
1 ½ cups almond flour
¼ cup coconut milk
½ teaspoon baking soda
1 teaspoon sea salt
¼ cup coconut oil
1 teaspoon palm sugar

<u>Method</u>

1. Mix almond flour, baking soda and salt together
2. In a separate bowl, whisk the two eggs until they are frothy. Then add coconut milk and whisk well.
3. Combine the dry ingredients with the wet ingredients and mix until a ball of dough forms. If the dough is becomes sticky add more almond flour.
4. Place the dough on a piece of parchment paper. Pat the dough down until it is about ½ inch thick.
5. Place another piece of parchment paper on top and place in the fridge for 30 minutes.
6. Whilst the dough is in fridge, take another two pieces of parchment paper. Place the hard coconut oil in between the paper and pound it until it is about 1/8 inch thick.
7. Remove the dough from the fridge and sprinkle a tiny bit of almond flour on the top of dough. Roll out the dough into a ¼ inch thick rectangle.
8. Spread the coconut oil on the top of the dough.

9. Now fold the dough into three. Fold the one long side in 1/3 of the way up the dough rectangle and fold the other side over the top of the folded flap.
10. Turn the dough from horizontal to vertical. And roll the dough again until it is ¼ inch thick.
11. Repeat folding and rolling action another 4 times.
12. Once that is done, cover with parchment paper again and place in fridge for 1 hour.
13. Preheat the oven to 450°F.
14. Take the dough out of the fridge and cut it into 9 equal squares. Then cut each square diagonally so that you have two triangles from each square (making 18 pieces).
15. Carefully roll each triangle (starting from the long side) into a croissant shape.
16. Place each on onto a well-greased baking tray and curve the croissant till it is in a 'C' shape.
17. Brush the egg white over each croissant and place in the oven to bake for 10 min or till they have become golden brown.
18. Allow to cool before serving.
19. These are too amazing for words!

*Note – to make my favorite Chocolate Croissants – simply place some dark chocolate pieces onto the triangles before you roll them up. When you bake them the chocolate will melt and become a decadent gooey treat that will have you salivating for seconds

Italian Pizza Dough
Yields: **1 pizza**

Ingredients

½ cup olive oil
½ cup water
½ cup almond flour
1 cup tapioca flour
1 teaspoon sea salt
1 teaspoon oregano
1 teaspoon garlic powder
1 teaspoon basil
1 large egg

Method

1. Preheat oven to 450°F
2. Mix the almond flour, tapioca, oregano, basil, garlic powder and salt together.
3. Mix water and oil together, then pour into dry ingredients and stir to combine.
4. Whisk an egg and add to the mixture. Mix well
5. Add more almond flour a tablespoon at a time (if necessary) until the mixture becomes a sticky dough.
6. Put the dough onto a lightly floured surface and knead it gently until it is more manageable to work with and no longer sticky.
7. Place the dough onto parchment paper and roll it out using a rolling pin.
8. Keep rolling until the dough is about 12 inches wide.
9. Place the parchment paper with the dough on it into the oven.
10. Bake for 15 minutes or until dough turns light brown.
11. Add topping of your choice and enjoy your delicious pizza.

Naan Bread
Yields: **1 loaf**

<u>Ingredients</u>

½ cup almond flour
½ cup tapioca flour
¼ cup olive oil
¼ cup coconut milk
4 eggs
4 tablespoons ground flax seeds
1 teaspoon apple cider vinegar
½ teaspoon salt
Coconut oil for frying

<u>Method</u>

1. Place all the ingredients into a bowl and mix everything together until it is well combined (the dough must not be too thick or too runny).
2. Melt 1 tablespoon of coconut oil in a non-stick pan, over a medium high heat.
3. Pour about 3 tablespoons of batter into the pan.
4. Gently tap down the batter to help it spread all over the bottom of the pan.
5. Cook for about 2 min before turning over.
6. Cook till the outside is slightly brown on both sides.
7. Allow to cool before eating.
8. Scrumptious as part of a Paleo Indian feast!

Conclusion

Thank you again for purchasing this book!

I hope it was able to help you to have a more complete and well-rounded Paleo lifestyle. There is nothing you have to ever be deprived of, because there are Paleo alternatives to all your favorites if you just know where to look!

The next step is to beat a hasty path to your nearest health store/supermarket and stock up the ingredients needed to bake delectable, scrumptious, mouth-watering breads!

Finally, if you enjoyed this book, please take the time to share your thoughts and post a review on Amazon. It'd be greatly appreciated!

Thank you and good luck!

Lucy Fast

Check out some of the other Yummy books in my Paleo Diet Solution Series!!

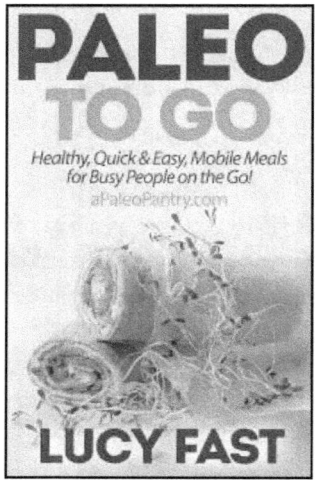

http://www.amazon.com/dp/B00HH1GBLC

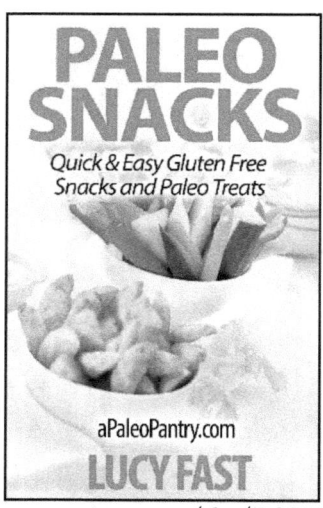

http://www.amazon.com/dp/B00IKYDUNW

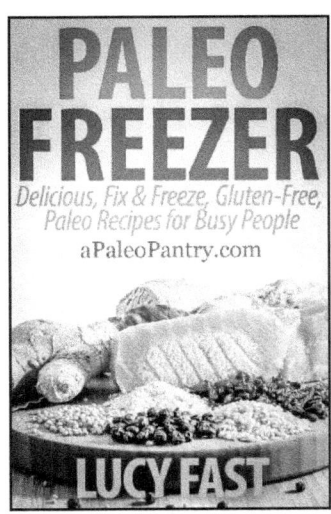

http://www.amazon.com/dp/B00HRMZΞ28

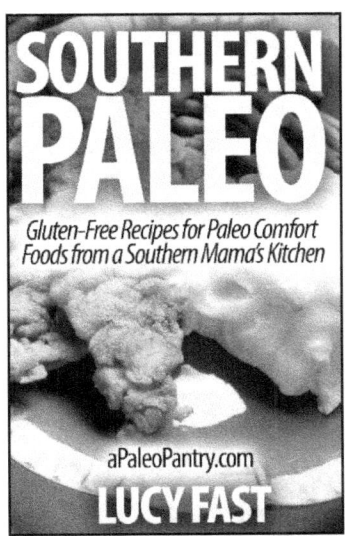

http://www.amazon.com/dp/B00HYKJCZ8

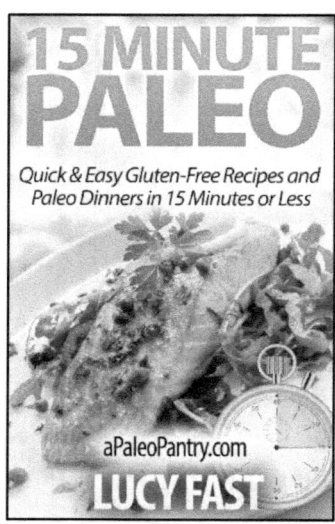

http://www.amazon.com/dp/B00I17R1ZQ

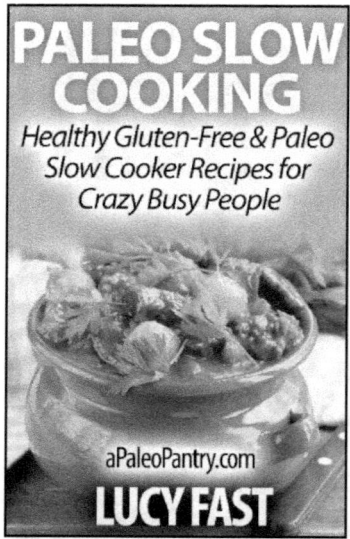

http://www.amazon.com/dp/B00I64CRQW

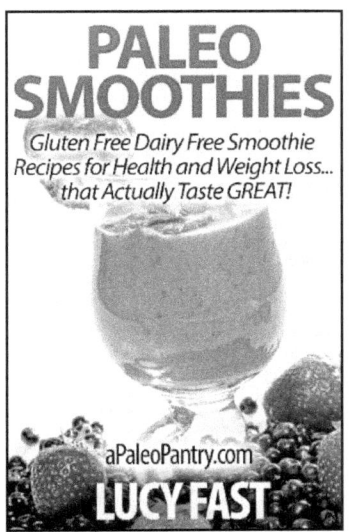

http://www.amazon.com/dp/B00ICYALXC

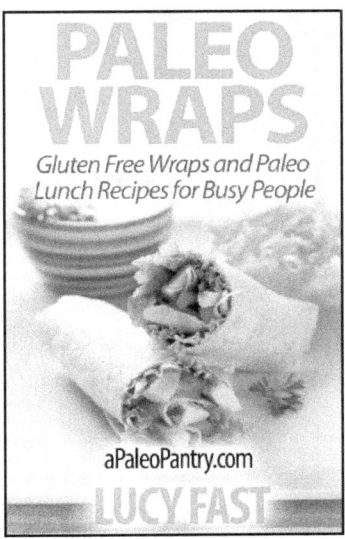

http://www.amazon.com/dp/B00IIHKA84

www.ingramcontent.com/pod-product-compliance
Lightning Source LLC
Chambersburg PA
CBHW060223290526
45789CB00003B/1392